CAREER AS A

PERSONAL TRAINER

FITNESS AND HEALTH EDUCATION

DO YOU THINK THAT EARNING A LIVING from your love for exercise is a stretch? It's not.

Careers in fitness are one of the fastest-growing segments of the US job market, and leading the way are personal trainers. In fact, the ranks of personal trainers have jumped by almost 50 percent over the last 10 years, and there is no sign of this job growth slowing up any time soon.

Young and old, men and women, people of all income levels are signing up for fitness classes and personal training sessions at an ever-increasing rate. With obesity being blamed for many of the health problems that people face today, thousands of people throughout the nation are determined to shed their extra weight. These people are turning to personal trainers to assist them in reaching that goal.

Reality television shows like *The Biggest Loser* have proven that no matter how overweight people are, they can slim down and learn how to stay fit with the aid of a knowledgeable personal trainer. Those who are already in good physical shape and want to stay that way also pay personal trainers to fine tune their exercise routines and provide expertise on the latest fitness trends. Athletes, dancers, rock singers, actors, and others whose professional careers rely on being in shape, retain personal trainers to keep them in peak form. Corporations bring in personal trainers to help top executives stay at their physical best. Today, more than ever before, the emphasis is maintaining good health by exercising and eating properly, and personal trainers can provide valuable insights in both these areas.

Fitness is a service industry. Every client is different, every client needs an individualized exercise program. Being a personal trainer is not a job that can be taken over by automation or outsourced to another country. This is work that needs to be done face to face, and your clients come to rely on your services. You become an important part of their weekly routine, and you tweak their fitness programs as they go through life.

Outstanding personal trainers can keep their clients for many years. When your clients look and feel good, you are rewarded. The job takes discipline and dedication. Personal trainers have to stay focused and must keep their clients motivated.

You are working with people one-on-one. You are in charge of their exercise regimens, and that makes being a personal trainer a results-oriented job. Whether they love to exercise or don't, your clients want to look in the mirror and be happy with what they see. If they aren't, they may not continue working out with you.

Successful personal trainers don't let their clients slack off. That means pushing clients to reach new fitness goals during every workout session, even though there are going to be days they just don't want to exercise. Each time you take on a client, you are putting your reputation on the line. With every success, the demand for your services grows, along with increased earnings.

WHAT YOU CAN DO NOW

MOST PEOPLE WHO BECOME PERSONAL trainers develop their passion for fitness and living a healthy lifestyle at an early age. They usually start out by learning about exercise and maintaining a proper diet so they can accomplish personal goals, like losing weight, building muscle mass, increasing strength and stamina, or just staying in superior shape and feeling better overall.

Taking courses on exercise and nutrition is a great introduction to the world of physical fitness. These courses are often offered at local YMCA-YWCAs, hospitals, gyms, and health clubs. By using this information to put together a fitness and dietary regimen for yourself, you will, in essence, become your first client.

Learning what it takes to keep yourself motivated to stick with the program will give you valuable insights that you can use throughout your career to keep your clients' enthusiasm at a high level. Reaching your fitness goals, and realizing the hard work it took to achieve your objectives, will become a great source of inspiration for you, and for your future clients as well.

Through your own workouts, you establish a fitness philosophy. You understand that staying fit takes commitment and follow-through, and ultimately becomes a way of life. Recognizing how you feel and the changes your body is going through as you are getting in shape provides you with a perspective on how clients will feel as they experience the same thing. Everything you do in your own fitness life is laying the groundwork for your future as a personal trainer.

HISTORY OF THE CAREER

PHYSICAL FITNESS IS TRENDY TODAY. However, it is also part of ancient history.

There is evidence that people followed a systematic exercise regimen as far back as 3600 BC, in China, Egypt, and Mesopotamia. By the sixth century BC, strength training, including weight lifting, was popular in ancient Greece, and civilization's battle to keep off those extra pounds was officially under way.

In these ancient times, many writers recorded the training methods of the armies of the world, noting the importance placed on muscular strength and conditioning.

British knights in medieval times had squires (perhaps some of the earliest personal trainers) who helped them work out and stay in superior condition, always ready to do battle. Shows of strength were an entertainment favorite in the Middle Ages, and the stars of these shows always had someone in their entourage to oversee their workouts and training.

In more modern times, professional strongmen would travel throughout the United States in the 1800s, dazzling audiences with their amazing physiques and putting on shows of death-defying muscular feats. Just seeing these strongmen perform would get youngsters excited about exercise and strength training.

There was a drawback to these exhibitions. They left the impression with the general public that working out was just about building huge muscles. The health and fitness aspect of exercise, not aiming for a bulging physique, was mostly overlooked. As a result, in the United States in the early 1900s, fitness training acquired a cult status. It was very popular with bodybuilders, but failed to attract the majority of the adult population.

That all changed when a fitness visionary entered the scene in the 1930s. Jack LaLanne, who is regarded as the father of the modern-day physical fitness movement, pioneered the personalized exercise program. He urged people in every walk of life, at every age, including children, to get off the couch and work their muscles, at least a little bit, every day. For many, this developed into a daily exercise routine.

LaLanne designed individual fitness plans tailored to the needs and goals of each of his clients, a bold concept when he started his health spa in 1936. At LaLanne's spa in Oakland, California, fitness buffs found a gym, a juice bar, and a health food store. The combination was unique, but LaLanne believed that both strenuous daily workouts and good nutrition were critical for overall good health.

LaLanne's health spa became the prototype for other fitness and health clubs around the country, and the exercise guru himself became well known in the San Francisco Bay Area for the results his workouts and wellness philosophy were achieving for his clients. In 1951, a local television station in San Francisco asked LaLanne to bring his jumping jacks and push-ups to the airwaves.

Using simple, everyday items, like chairs and broomsticks, that everyone could find around the house, he showed people how easy it was to get in shape and stay in shape, right in the comfort of their own home.

The show was broadcast nationwide starting in 1959, making LaLanne a celebrity and propelling exercise and nutrition into the mainstream. The show aired weekdays for more than 30 years, and millions of viewers got into the habit of setting aside time every day to exercise.

LaLanne's secret to success on the airwaves was that he made it personal. He seemed to be able to go beyond the frame of the television set and reach viewers on a one-to-one basis, as if he were right there in their homes. He was everyone's personal trainer. LaLanne paved the way for future TV fitness experts, like Richard Simmons, to bring their training methods to people everywhere through the magic of television.

Exercise also got a boost in the early 1960s from President John F. Kennedy, who called physical fitness a defining principle of his administration. Children were a prime focus of President Kennedy's fitness program. A school curriculum was developed to improve fitness for youngsters on all grade levels. Many of those children carried their early lessons into adulthood, maintaining a workout routine and going to a gym regularly.

The fitness movement surged in the late 1970s, when many professional exercise specialists in large cities started opening clubs geared to the needs of the individual. Fitness enthusiasts loved the one-on-one attention they were getting, and the personal trainer became a permanent part of the fitness industry.

In the 1980s, so many people were hiring personal trainers to help them slim down and tone up that it caught the attention of the news media. The headlines boosted the public's interest in these fitness miracle workers even more.

Exercise mania swelled the membership rolls of gyms and health clubs everywhere. Those who wanted to get away from the crowds asked the personal trainers they worked with at the gym if they would make house calls. Workout expertise started being delivered to America's front door.

Soon, some of the more popular personal trainers, like Kathy Smith, Jullian Michaels, and movie star Jane Fonda, were writing books and putting out exercise tapes, so they could reach millions more people. It seemed that the public could not get enough information on ways to stay fit.

There are so many fitness celebrities today that there is even a list of The 100 Most Influential People in Health and Fitness, with links to their websites and TV shows. Check it out here

http://greatist.com/most-influential-health-fitness-people

Exercise and fitness have become big business and a great career opportunity.

WHERE YOU WILL WORK

GYMS AND HEALTH CLUBS ARE JUST two of the locations where personal trainers are employed. Naturally, these facilities have everything trainers need to help clients accomplish their fitness goals. Personal trainers can also be found flexing their muscles outside the traditional gym in other segments of the working and leisure world. Many large corporations have fully equipped gyms right in their own headquarters to help employees stay in shape without leaving the premises. To enhance the workout experience and gear it more to the needs of particular individuals, some of these companies employ personal trainers on staff and on site. Employees can consult them to help develop a personalized fitness program.

Hospitals and colleges also have personal trainers on their campuses to work with employees and students who want professional input when it comes to developing and sticking with an exercise and wellness program. With health insurers putting an emphasis on preventive care, this is one of the ways that large organizations can show that they are taking steps to help people stay healthy and in top physical condition. This, in turn, helps lower health insurance premiums.

Cruise ships, resorts, and health spas have personal trainers available for patrons who want to take advantage of a one-on-one fitness experience while on vacation. Having personal trainers on hand is a strong selling point used to help promote these venues. There is the added bonus for personal trainers: these vacation destinations are often located in exotic locales, making for some plush workplaces in pleasurable climates.

Personal trainers who work with professional athletes might work at a team's training center. For athletes involved in more individual sports, like ice-skating, skiing, or swimming, personal trainers may operate at an ice rink, at a ski resort, or even poolside.

Going where they are needed is part of the job description for personal trainers. That means that if their methods and techniques have proven successful, these fitness experts can find themselves getting job offers anywhere in the world. Trainers may even travel with clients whose work takes them from one far-off location to another. Many movie stars have been known to take their personal trainers with them on movie shoots.

You do not have to be a fitness guru to the stars to find work. People in every walk of life are hiring personal trainers. These trainers do their job where those who hire them are most comfortable, which might be at home, in a park, or at the gym.

Personal trainers with a large client base often have a fully equipped small portable gym of their own for individual workouts. Clients can have personalized sessions and work out in the privacy of their own homes. It's a convenient, comfortable, and familiar atmosphere for clients, where they can easily relax after a strenuous workout. Making house calls is a plus for personal trainers as well. They get some downtime between fitness sessions, and a chance to unwind both physically and mentally, while they commute from one location to another. They also don't have to share the fees with an employer who pays for the expenses of operating a health club.

THE WORK YOU WILL DO

AS A PERSONAL TRAINER, THE FITNESS needs of your clients, and how they can reach their goals, are your primary concern. Unless you are employed full time in a health club, you are also a businessperson and you have to run your business successfully, doing everything from maintaining financial records to promoting your services.

There is plenty to do when you take on this job, and you'll get a pretty good workout yourself. When you are working with someone, you have to give that person your undivided attention. You are paid to provide personalized service, and if you don't deliver that kind of service, you won't be successful.

When you first get new clients, you have to take the time to really get to know each of them. Learn about their careers, their families, their hobbies, their likes and dislikes. That will help you design a workout program that fits each of them the best, while establishing a solid rapport with them.

The job of putting together an exercise routine is similar to that of a choreographer. The workout has to have a flow, with one exercise transitioning into another. The program must be challenging yet enjoyable, filled with exercises that will have an impact. It is a creative process because you strive to develop exercise routines for clients that will hold their interest.

Variety is often the key. You start every program with a warm-up, end each one with a cool-down and stretching, and include cardiovascular, resistance, and core strengthening in every workout. These are the elements of a solid exercise routine.

The degree of difficulty varies with each of your clients, and depends upon their individual needs and goals. You teach clients how to run through their own programs. Most of the time you will be there to help and guide them, but they should be able to do the whole routine on their own. That involves showing the client how to warm up and cool down, and for how long.

Teaching the principles of resistance, core strengthening, and cardiovascular training is part of your job. You must be adamant about discouraging clients from taking shortcuts and doing sloppy workouts when you are not around. You are constantly stressing the discipline to do the workouts properly and in full.

Everybody has a different lifestyle. Some people are busier than others, work longer hours, travel constantly, are more driven. There are age differences and overall physical health to be taken into account.

Doing a health screening is part of the initial work you will do when you first take on a client. You must know about any medical conditions a person might have now, as well as past injuries or surgeries. Finding out about any allergies a person has and medications being taken, is also part of the screening, as is a complete family medical history. An exercise history of the client is useful as well. This information helps you determine the risk factors and special needs of each individual.

People have to let you into their lives. That is the only way for you to develop a fitness program that will truly work for them. Building trust is essential. Personal trainers become confidants to many clients simply because they go through so many life changes with these people. It is the nature of the job.

If you have clients long enough, you may see them as they switch jobs, get married, have children, move, suffer losses, and have illnesses. All these circumstances and many more spark reactions that affect exercise routines and eating habits. Knowing what is going on in a client's life helps prepare you to respond to the situation.

You have to set the tone. Some people might want to conquer the world. Others would rather take things more slowly – perhaps too slowly. The personal trainer is the voice of reason. You know the right way to establish goals and keep everything balanced.

From your experience, you know that failing to reach goals, especially early on in the fitness experience, can be very discouraging and cause clients to suffer an emotional setback. So the goals you set at first may be a bit easy to reach, but you raise the bar much higher as you go along.

Discussing exercise routines with clients is very important. It is your job to establish a good line of communications with your clients. Invite them to be part of the process by encouraging them to make suggestions and ask questions. One way to keep clients involved is by soliciting their input. If a client feels that a goal is too easy to reach, bump it up a notch. Show clients that you value their opinions.

Never underestimate your role as a motivator. Everyone is motivated differently, and you have to figure out what gets each of your clients going. The feedback you give is positive; any criticism is constructive.

People will pay you to work with them three or more times a week because they need that push to work out. They won't or can't get themselves to exercise on their own, so they need you there to oversee what they are doing.

You have to be energized every time you meet. Whether it is at the gym or in the person's home, you are always ready to go. When you are around, there is no quitting. You are a source of encouragement and inspiration. Teaching your clients how to muscle through difficult times is why you are on the job. In fitness training there are ups and downs, and clients have to be able to handle both the good and the bad.

Personal trainers monitor everything that is going on with their clients. They make sure exercises are being done properly and are achieving the desired results. Tweaking fitness programs as you go along is what you are there for. Making those adjustments as soon as they are needed keeps the training program on track.

Part of your job is to teach your clients about nutrition and how to maintain a healthy diet. This should be a component of any fitness program. Getting people to eat healthier can be more difficult than getting them to exercise. Unhealthy temptations are all around, and people tend to grab whatever food is available when they are busy and on the run.

Dietary changes are a matter of breaking ingrained habits. As with the exercise regimen you establish for them, people will look to you for leadership and understanding as they take this dietary leap of faith.

Keeping accurate records of the exercises performed at each session and the intensity level is important to tracking progress. This information should be recorded as it happens to make sure it is precise. It is also good to have these notes in the event that a client suffers an injury, so you know exactly what transpired during each workout.

Preventing client burnout is a major issue for personal trainers. Client burnout is one of the main reasons personal trainers lose good, regular, long-term customers. One of the first signs of this problem is appointment cancellations. You might also notice that a client is agitated, seems depressed, uninterested, or unable to complete workouts. Jumping in and getting to the root of the problem will help you get your client's workouts back on track.

Many times, burnout can be traced to overtraining. Exercise has many health benefits, but sometimes you end up with too much of a good thing. Maybe a client has to step back a bit, or you have to add some other activities, like yoga or Pilates, on certain days to vary the workout and keep it engaging.

Perhaps there are just not enough aspects of the routine that clients enjoy anymore, and you have to adjust the workout to reignite their interest. A location change may be in order and help freshen things up. Clients who like to do all their workouts at home may get reenergized by going to the gym, exercising in the park, or taking a swim at the local pool after going through their exercise routine. Being able to work through problems like burnout successfully is what distinguishes great personal trainers.

Always have a few surprises in your repertoire. Surprises are just that – the unexpected that happens every once in a while. They keep your clients on their toes, can go a long way toward preventing burnout and boredom, and are just plain fun. In other words, you might want to spice things up every once in a while.

As an example, some personal trainers know people at the training facilities of professional sports teams. These trainers can get their clients in every once in a while to see how the pros work out. The clients see the equipment the athletes use and the paces their trainers put them through, and sometimes even work out with these pros for a few minutes or more. What an uplifting experience – to see how hard these athletes have to work, that it just doesn't come naturally to them. It is reinvigorating for your clients and gives them a new perspective on what it takes to stay in top form and condition.

Another important aspect of your job is knowing about the latest information and trends in the fitness world. That keeps you at the top of your game and allows your clients to stay on the cutting edge. You don't want your clients to give you breaking news from the fitness industry – you want to be the first to tell them about it. That involves everything from the latest exercise theory to the newest equipment.

Taking classes in person or online, attending seminars and workshops, reading professional training and nutrition magazines and journals, and talking with other trainers and people in the exercise world, are all measures to keep you informed and updated. Even though you have been involved in the industry for a while, you can never stop learning.

When you are not in the gym or on the exercise mat, you must devote some time to running your business. Even if you work full time at a gym or a health club, you have to set a goal of building and maintaining your client base. You want to keep your clients for years, while adding new clients from time to time. Ideally, the time to establish your client base is when you are just breaking into the business. Once you start taking on clients, you want to keep them in the fold, while pacing yourself as you add new ones.

To build a solid client base, you must develop some marketing skills. Knowing how to sell your services, promote your strengths, and spark interest in what you can do to help people reach their fitness goals, are integral to succeeding as a personal trainer.

Properly evaluating your clients will help you provide the type of service they desire. Know which clients want you to push them hard and which ones respond better when you are a bit more laid back. Being able to get results both ways is one of the keys to success.

Never take any of your clients for granted. Their concerns are your concerns. You need to make each of your clients feel as though he or she is the most important, if not the only, person you are working with. Mastering that ability can set the tone for your entire business.

Networking inside and outside of the fitness industry should be on your agenda. Networking within the industry gives you the opportunity to meet and get to know the movers and shakers in the business and become one yourself. Networking outside the fitness world with other business owners and people in your community keeps your name front and center, and opens the door to a possible client pool, which is always a plus.

I Am a Personal Trainer With My Own

Gym "I own my own private gym and many people come here to work out. I am a personal trainer. Not all of the people who come here need or want the services of a personal trainer and that's fine; one is not contingent on the other.

I work as a personal trainer with people who want one-on-one training. For some clients, I work with them in their own homes. The advantage of the gym is that there is very extensive equipment here.

Some people have exercise equipment in their homes. Others will ask me to set up a gym for them in their home, and there are those people who want to work with as little equipment as possible. I can work with things that are around the house, like stairs, chairs, and coffee tables. I even bring some small equipment with me, like mats, dumbbells, and exercise bands.

Sometimes people who are not into exercise just can't get motivated to get to the gym. They miss, cancel, or come late to appointments. There is less of that when you go to people's homes. They are usually already there. Many of them work at home, they have greater flexibility, it is convenient, and the comfort level is high – no worries about being embarrassed or looking silly.

Even though I have the gym, I like working with clients in their own homes. I think when people call you to work with them on a fitness program at home, they are going to follow through. They have made the decision to stick with it. Not that I don't have serious clients in the gym, but they tend to be younger people or someone who has been into exercise for a while.

The calls I get from people who want in-home services tend to come from middle-aged to older folks, who have not worked out for a while and really need to get into shape. It has taken a lot for them to take this step, and they might not be ready to work out in a public setting. If they have to do that, they probably will not go ahead with it. Sometimes you don't have as much space in a person's home as you would like, but you work with it. The most important thing is to listen to the clients. What are their concerns and what do they want to accomplish? Then you design a workout program that fits those needs.

11

I also work with nutrition. I think eating properly helps people get in shape and stay that way. I never lose sight of the fact that the path to getting fit may require breaking some bad habits, and that takes time. It can be a slow process that requires a great deal of patience on your part. It is not going to happen until a client realizes the benefits associated with breaking those bad habits. Once that occurs, most people can't understand why they didn't do it sooner. Those breakthroughs can be very rewarding for you and your clients."

I Am a Personal Trainer for a College
Sports Program "I never really planned on working with competitive athletes. I started out working in a gym, as most personal trainers do. I then began developing a steady group of regular clients.

Most of my clients were people who wanted to get in shape. My clients were not really very overweight, though some did need to drop a few pounds. Most just felt they would feel better by following a regular exercise routine and having a healthier diet. Interestingly, I found that none of them really knew how to get started on this quest, and that's where I came in.

I live in a town with a medium-sized college nearby. One day a football player from the school who had heard about me stopped by and started asking me questions about strength training and conditioning. I knew a lot about that, since I was a wrestler in high school and college. The player's main concern was that he kept getting nagging injuries that really slowed his game. Many young athletes have this problem because they don't get involved in what many doctors now refer to as 'prehabilitation.'

Prehab is basically strength training and conditioning to avoid injury. So, prehab is designed to avoid rehab. Many nagging injuries happen because athletes exercise one part of the body vigorously, and neglect another. For instance, people work their stomach muscles, but completely overlook exercising their lower back, making it a prime target for an injury – sometimes a rather serious one.

You study the training procedures of athletes and see what they are failing to do to strengthen the entire body, especially those vulnerable areas they do not think about. They may assume nothing can be done to avoid an injury. Then you draw up an exercise program to address those needs. That's what I did for this particular player.

A common problem is ankle sprains, especially in football. They happen all the time, and athletes think you can't do anything to stop them from occurring, but you can. Building strong leg muscles is one of the ways ankle sprains can be prevented. Most athletes don't work on strengthening their lower leg muscles every day, if at all.

After I started working with this one player and was having success, other players came to see me. The players were doing this on their own; the school was not involved yet. One of the players must have mentioned the work I was doing to one of the coaches, and I was called in for a meeting with the entire football coaching staff.

After several rather long meetings, where I explained my work with the players and my theories about preventing injuries before they happened, the school offered to pay me to come in and work with athletes on a one-on-one basis.

I started with the football team. It was voluntary for the athletes; no one was forced to use my services, but I was there for them by appointment. Many of the football players took advantage of the program. Athletes on other school teams also started seeking out my advice.

You really have to be knowledgeable in all areas of exercise science to work in the field of strength training and conditioning on the college or pro sports level. In fact, many colleges and pro sports teams these days look for someone with a bachelor's degree, or even a master's in exercise science or a related subject, to do the kind of work I do with these athletes.

You are measured on how well you keep a team up and running. No one expects that there will be no injuries at all, but coaches do expect to see a noticeable drop in those constant nagging injuries. Doing that justifies having you around. There is pressure in this job because the success of others rides on what you do. Some major colleges and pro teams have strength and conditioning trainers on staff; some have even elevated the job to a coaching status. Others just keep personal trainers on as consultants. Then there are those players who prefer to work with a personal trainer of their own choosing, someone who focuses solely on their individual conditioning needs."

I Am a Personal Trainer in a Corporate

Setting "When a large corporation in town decided to build a gym within their headquarters building, I was called in to work with employees who wanted to consult with a personal trainer. At the time, I was already the personal trainer for two of the executives who worked at the company, so they knew my work and recommended me. I liked this situation very much because it gave me an instant client base and a chance to work with people with varying fitness and wellness issues.

Many of the people I work with in this setting never knew exactly what a personal trainer could do for them. I think the thing that surprises people the most is that they really do not know how to exercise properly. I think once they learn the right way to exercise and see some of the benefits of it, they get comfortable with it and even look forward to working out. They feel better and it has an impact on their life both at work and at home. The remark I hear most from people who train with me is 'I have so much more energy.'

People often fear exercise. They think they will get hurt or can only be successful if they develop six-pack abs. I always stress the fact that sometimes you can get hurt because you don't exercise. You don't use your muscles, and one day you get up to do something and you pull a muscle you haven't used for years. So, you actually avoid getting hurt by staying loose and keeping active.

The first thing I try to do is make the experience fun for them. I try to design an exercise program they will enjoy. Nothing too difficult – I always start out slow, especially with people who have not exercised in a long time. I try to teach them something about the exercises so they know what they are doing and why.

I want people to feel they can't wait to get to the gym, to get away from the desk and the computer. I show people how they can relieve stress and tension through exercise, and actually relax.

I take clients by appointment, and while I usually work one-on-one, if two friends want to partner for a session, I never balk at that. Sometimes that becomes a friendly competition and they push each other. I don't see the same clients every day, though I encourage my clients to come to the corporate gym every day and work on what we did during our private sessions. I try to get them into a daily routine, even if we only get together once a week. It could be my imagination, but I see a more robust workforce here."

PERSONAL QUALIFICATIONS

AS A PERSONAL TRAINER, YOU ARE A motivator, coach, teacher, and friend. You will be introducing people to a new way of life and, in the process, changing their lives for the better. Clients look for a trainer who is energetic and exudes confidence, a role model for them to follow as they embark on this journey.

Personal trainers have to be experts in fitness techniques, and be able to share that knowledge. That means having a total understanding of anatomy, exercise physiology, and nutrition. It is not enough to instruct a client to do something – you have to explain why you are telling the client to do it. Having excellent communications skills is very important in this field. Clients want to know why you are recommending certain exercises for them to do, and what will be accomplished by doing them. By clearly explaining the particular exercises you choose for a person's workout regimen, and discussing the overall exercise program in full, you keep the client involved in the process, and that is vital for success.

You need to take the time to demonstrate how to do an exercise properly. This is where you utilize your teaching skills. People think they know how to exercise, but most don't. You have to show them how each movement is done, talk about how it feels as the muscle tightens and stretches, and make sure clients are doing the exercise the right way. At the very least, there is nothing gained when an exercise is not done right. At worst, doing an exercise the wrong way could lead to serious injury.

Reaching fitness goals requires discipline. To teach discipline to your clients, you have to have it yourself. Clients must learn how to resist the temptations of fast food, large portion sizes, and skipping workouts when you are not around. You have to help clients break bad habits and replace them with healthy choices. This takes patience.

Changes do not occur overnight. It could take time for a client to completely accept your fitness philosophy. If you give up easily, your clients will, too. You go through the ups and downs with them, encouraging clients to exceed even their own expectations.

Leadership qualities are necessary as you influence, guide, and direct the people you are working with on a daily basis. You have to be able to instill the desire in your clients to make the changes necessary for them to feel and look better.

Being creative is imperative, too. Exercise programs are not a one-size-fits-all proposition. You have to be able to design workouts that suit the needs of each client. You have to find ways to prevent their routines from becoming stale and boring.

Building incentives into each of the programs you design is a must. Making sure your clients stay focused falls back on you. You must keep your clients interested in sticking with the program, and motivate them even when they feel that progress is slow. Offering words of encouragement and knowing just how much to push each client are both part of your game plan.

Maintaining a high level of professionalism at all times is of the utmost importance. You arrive on time for appointments, dress neatly, and treat everyone with respect.

ATTRACTIVE FEATURES

A PERSONAL TRAINER TRULY HELPS people. When people lose weight and adopt a healthier lifestyle as a result of your intervention, you feel a true sense of accomplishment. In many cases you are helping people get their lives back and be more active. You can derive great satisfaction from seeing people become fit, trim, and healthy as a result of your planning and guidance.

The opportunity for success stories is unlimited. In reality, by working with just one person, you can have an impact on an entire family.

Helping people achieve fitness goals they have been unable to reach for years motivates you all the time. It becomes a driving force that spurs you on to do your job better. It makes your job meaningful and worthwhile.

You have the knowledge that you are teaching people life lessons that will remain with them for years. The chance to interact with people who need your valuable insights makes you an integral part of their lives.

You are doing something meaningful in a field you believe in. As a personal trainer, you already know the benefits of exercise and proper nutrition. You practice what you preach and maintain a healthy lifestyle. You are promoting something that is important to you and plays a significant role in your own life.

As a personal trainer, there is no sitting behind a desk all day. This is a job where you are active all the time. It never gets dull. You have a chance to see the results of your work each day.

Developing your own training methods and techniques, then using them with your clientele, is one of the rewards of this job. You are free to draw on the fitness philosophies you have put together through the years to structure a successful workout and nutrition program for your clients.

16

There is an opportunity to make a name for yourself in the fitness field by finding a niche. You can choose to limit your work to senior citizens, young people, or athletes, for example. Your focus might be on people who are rehabbing an injury or battling eating disorders. When you specialize, you can get known for your work in a particular area, and then you can market your services to that target audience. Many clients look for fitness experts with a reputation for having success working with one age group or another, or helping people with special needs.

If you enjoy being your own boss, working as a personal trainer provides you with that option. Many personal trainers run their own business, with the freedom to choose their own clients, make policy, and set their own schedule. In other words, you make all the decisions, including setting fees. This gives you a great deal of flexibility.

Personal trainers whose methods have proven to be successful are often able to parlay their one-on-one work with clients into TV shows, books and videos, opening up a new stream of income.

UNATTRACTIVE ASPECTS

A CAREER AS A PERSONAL TRAINER IS not all about fitness. If you are in business for yourself, you have to be able to sell your services. Getting people who have never trained with you excited about what you have to offer is essential in building a client list. You will have to do marketing and networking. Some people are uncomfortable promoting themselves, but it's essential to surviving in this field.

In order to be financially successful, you will have to grow your client base consistently. This means taking some time away from working with clients to meet with people, talk about your services, and try to get them to workout with you. In addition, you must attend to some mundane business matters – like bookkeeping, banking, and taxes.

Working for a gym or a health club relieves you of the business responsibilities, but you are locked into someone else's rules, policies, scheduling, and to some degree, training philosophy. Your earnings will also be limited by your salary, stable but with little upside potential.

Working with people can be frustrating, especially if they are reluctant to give your methods a try. Though clients might say they are serious about losing weight or adopting a healthy lifestyle, when it comes to actually doing it, that might be a different story.

Clients might work out or eat healthy when you are around, but are they committed enough to stick with the program with no supervision? If they don't, and if they fail to reach their fitness goals, they might blame you, rather than admitting that they slacked off.

You might find that a particular client is just not willing to do what it takes to make a fitness program successful, and you have to part ways with that person. Severing ties with any client is difficult – you have a vested interest in that person. Even if the client was never really committed to the program, you still feel as though you failed in some way.

Going into this field, you have to realize that working a normal schedule is out of the question. Many of your clients have jobs and will probably want to work out before or after work. Some will prefer having you work with them on weekends. On weekdays, you will probably have early-morning sessions as well as evening and night appointments. There will be downtime during the rest of the day. Weekends will probably be heavily booked all day. Working while most people are off requires an adjustment in your lifestyle that you will have to make. Flexibility is required. As with any service-oriented business, people will cancel appointments and will want to reschedule, so you have to be able to fit them in.

There is always a risk that a client may suffer an injury during a workout and blame you for it. This can be unpleasant, especially if it results in a lawsuit. Insurance companies do offer liability coverage for personal trainers. This is a business matter you will have to deal with in order to protect yourself from any legal liability.

EDUCATION AND TRAINING

YOU DON'T HAVE TO GET A COLLEGE education to become a personal trainer, but more people today are deciding to enter the fitness field prepared with a bachelor's degree. Some even go on to earn a master's degree.

People seeking the services of a personal trainer want the best-qualified person they can find, and having a college degree certainly helps give you an edge in the competition for clients.

Prospective personal trainers who go to college can earn degrees in exercise science, exercise physiology, physical education, or kinesiology. They take courses in health, nutrition, psychology, and sports medicine as well. The more you know about the field, the better prepared you are to answer the difficult questions clients will ask you. You will be able to design effective exercise programs for clients with special needs, including senior citizens, people with disabilities, and those who want to build strength after recovering from an injury.

Having a solid educational background in exercise science and fitness also prepares you to consult with doctors, physical therapists, and other healthcare professionals, who might be working with one of your clients.

There are associate degrees offered in exercise science at community colleges across the country. Schools like Raritan Valley Community College in Branchburg, New Jersey; Three Rivers Community College in Norwich, Connecticut; Mesa Community College in Arizona; and Washtenaw Community College in Ann Arbor, Michigan, are among the many two-year schools with exercise science programs.

Another option is to earn a bachelor's degree in exercise science at a four-year college. In an exercise science curriculum, students study how the human body responds to fitness training. Neuromuscular function, cardiovascular physiology, and biochemical changes associated with exercises are some of the subject areas explored. Courses in diet, nutrition, and sports medicine are also offered as part of the exercise science degree program at many colleges.

The University of Tampa in Florida, and Mercy College in Dobbs Ferry, New York both offer a bachelor's degree program in exercise science. The University of Massachusetts in Amherst confers BAs in exercise science, exercise and health science, as well as fitness instruction and management. West Virginia University in Morgantown offers a bachelor's degree in exercise physiology, as well as a master's and PhD in the subject. Baylor University in Waco, Texas, also has bachelor's and master's degree programs in exercise physiology.

In Provo, Utah, Brigham Young University's Department of Exercise Science has a series of bachelor's degree programs in three disciplines: exercise science, exercise and wellness, and athletic training. Brigham Young students can also earn a master's degree in exercise science, exercise physiology and athletic training, and a PhD in exercise physiology.

There are also many programs in kinesiology, the scientific study of human movement. Four-year schools, like the University of Minnesota in Minneapolis, Towson University in Maryland, and Kansas State University in Manhattan, award bachelor's degrees in kinesiology. Advanced degrees are also available. Baylor University, for instance, has a PhD in kinesiology.

For those who work full time and may not be able to attend classes in person on a regular basis, there are accredited online schools that have degree programs in exercise science. Those schools include Concordia University and Broadview University. Globe University/Minnesota School of Business has campuses throughout Minnesota with an online component. The school has a four-year health fitness specialist degree that was designed with the needs of personal trainers in mind.

Personal trainers never stop learning, so you should be committed to taking continuing education courses from reputable fitness associations throughout your career.

Whether you go to college or not, having a certification – or several of them – from well-respected organizations in the field is vital. Know as much as you can about any organization before getting certified by the group. The standards for certification should be rigorous and the organization should demand a certain amount of continuing education for you to keep your certification. Only seek out certifications by an organization that has been accredited by an unbiased third party, like the highly regarded National Organization for Competency Assurance (NOCA). Some groups that offer accreditation and award certifications to personal trainers are the American Council on Exercise (ACE), the National Strength and Conditioning Association (NSCA), the National Academy of Sports Medicine (NASM) and the American College of Sports Medicine. Read about the different certifications and get the one that suits your needs.

It is important for personal trainers to have certificates in CPR (cardiopulmonary resuscitation) and AED (automated external defibrillator).

Personal trainers do not have to be licensed at this time, but experts in the field believe that will change within the coming decade, and licensing will be required, most likely on the state level. That would actually be a good thing for the profession, since it will enhance the status of qualified trainers.

EARNINGS

THERE ARE MANY FACTORS THAT GO into determining the income of a personal trainer. One of the most important is your reputation. Personal trainers with a solid track record of success can command a higher rate than trainers who are just starting out in the field. Word-of-mouth recommendations are vital to boosting your client base, and as the demand for your services grows, so will your earnings. If there are more people who want your services, you can usually charge a higher rate.

Personal trainers in large urban areas, like New York City, Los Angeles, Chicago and Houston, for instance, have a bigger population pool looking for their services than fitness experts in rural areas, where working out might not be as popular. You have to consider what the competition in a particular geographical area is charging clients for similar services and how high the cost of living in that area is.

Generally speaking, personal trainers charge by the hour or by the session. Sometimes a wealthy client or a pro athlete will want you to devote several hours or even days just to them, and you can charge accordingly.

Hourly rates range from $25 an hour for trainers just starting out, to $125 or more for those well-established in the field. The average rate is about $65 an hour. Some trainers charge more for prime hours (early mornings, evenings) or on the weekend.

What you earn comes down to the amount of time you want to put in and how many clients you have. Personal trainers with a full client load can earn $75,000 or more a year. Those who acquire celebrity status – putting out videos and books, appearing on TV, and gaining a following online – can earn substantially more.

The services of a personal trainer are also available through a health club or gym on a per session basis. Personal trainers employed at health clubs or gyms receive a percentage of the fee paid by each client they have a session with at the facility. At these clubs and gyms, the sessions generally last one hour and cost about $75 per session. The personal trainer usually gets 40 percent of the fee, or $30. If clients decide to take out a membership at the club as a result of the work the personal trainer is doing with them, the trainer gets a commission, normally 15 to 20 percent for each one.

Yearly income for personal trainers who work in health clubs is based on how many clients they can get. Many of these trainers only work part time at a club, and therefore their salaries average about $30,000 a year. These trainers commonly have clients outside of the club as well, making additional income from those sessions.

The personal trainers who decide to pursue this career on a full-time basis try to get away from the clubs so they don't have to share fees. Working at the clubs is a starting point, the goal being either to get your own gym or to make house calls.

Some trainers have a rental arrangement with clubs and gyms. They pay for a block of time at the facility and then schedule client sessions there. They are not employees of the facility. Under this arrangement, personal trainers can see clients for as long as they want and set their own fees.

OPPORTUNITIES

WITH AMERICA'S WAISTLINE EXPANDing more than ever before, the need for personal trainers is growing with it. Obesity is always in the headlines and people are constantly being urged to finally make the commitment to lose weight. Seems like the advantages of living a healthy lifestyle are trumpeted everywhere these days, from the White House to the school room.

There are plenty of natural times throughout the year when people decide they want to take the plunge. New Year's is always popular for resolutions to lose weight. That is a perfect time for personal trainers to promote themselves and offer introductory rates to attract new clients.

As summer approaches, the warmer weather signals another surge in weight-loss efforts. People feel it is time to get in shape to don a bathing suit, so they can enjoy some fun in the sun.

Birthdays make many people take a hard look at themselves and choose to make a change for the better. News stories throughout the year about celebrities who have lost weight encourage even more people to try to take off the pounds.

Though the interest in fitness spikes at particular times of the year, there is never really a lull in the exercise and wellness business. That keeps you busy. Many people feel that being in top physical condition will help them live longer and be more productive, so they are always interested in what you have to offer. Since physical fitness is something foreign to most people, they turn to a professional to give them insight into the latest trends, both in exercise and nutrition.

Americans with a busy schedule love having a personal trainer come to their home to help them stay in shape. Having a personal trainer gives people the chance to talk about fitness and nutrition with someone they trust. They can exchange ideas about exercise programs, workout equipment, and healthy foods with an expert. Tweaking workout programs helps people avoid wasting time performing exercises that do not help them. Mostly, they just need someone to "make" them do it.

These are all services you can provide. As a fitness expert and personal trainer who does house calls, you are in great demand today. You can also help people who want to stay in shape but do not have the time to engage in lengthy exercise sessions every day. Working with busy corporate executives, you can devise high-impact daily exercise programs that give these people the maximum benefit in the shortest time possible. That can develop into a niche market for you.

Personal trainers play a vital role in the sports arena. One of the fastest-growing aspects of the fitness industry is personal trainers who work with athletes on all levels, from high school to pro sports. Teams are looking to personal trainers to help their players put together workout programs that will build strength and avoid injury. They want someone who can work with players on a one-to-one basis, giving them the individual attention they need. Athletes involved in individual sports, like running, swimming, gymnastics, and cycling, are looking to do the same thing.

Not all sports-related injuries are avoidable. In cases when an athlete suffers an injury, a personal trainer is summoned to help that athlete return to top form.

GETTING STARTED

YOU MAY BE IN GREAT SHAPE, BUT nobody is going to know just by looking at you that you're a personal trainer. You have to get the word out, and the best way to do that is to go where prospective clients are plentiful. That is why most personal trainers start their careers by working in gyms, spas, and health clubs.

Working in these venues gives young personal trainers, just starting out, a chance to learn the business. You can mingle with other experienced trainers, who can be a valuable resource for you. This gives you an opportunity to exchange ideas and concerns with people who have been in the business for a while, observe how they work with clients, and learn the tricks of the trade firsthand.

This experience will give you the time you need to establish yourself as a trainer. In addition, these clubs have top-notch equipment that clients can use. That spares you the expense of having to buy pricey workout equipment when you are just starting out.

There are several valuable lessons you will learn while on the job at a gym, spa, or health club. First of all, you'll find that these venues are competitive. All the personal trainers working there are trying to line up clients. Through some trial and error, and by watching some of the other trainers in action, you can hone your marketing skills and find out what works for you when trying to interest potential clients in your services.

How good are you at following up with people? Just because people say no to you today does not mean they won't be interested in hiring you sometime down the road. Do you have a plan to stay on their radar? Did you send a note thanking them for meeting with you?

Consider sending out monthly e-mails with fitness and nutrition tips to prospective clients who have met with you but have not hired you yet. These early years when you are just starting out in the business will give you the opportunity to experiment with your sales pitch and your follow-up to see what works and what doesn't. By doing so, you can fine-tune your approach.

Among the vitally important insights you will gain by working in a gym, spa, or health club early in your career is learning how to work and deal with the variety of personalities you come across in these venues. Working with people with varying degrees of expertise in the world of fitness – from the novice to the very experienced – is what will make this job challenging.

Structuring an exercise program for someone who has never stepped on a treadmill will be easy for you. For people who have worked out for years and want to refresh their program, you will have to be a bit more creative. You will come across those who struggle to make the smallest accomplishments, and those who reach new goals with ease. Learning how to make the adjustments necessary so you can maximize the success you have with each of your clients is what will eventually set you apart in this field.

ASSOCIATIONS

- **National Federation of Personal Trainers (NFPT)**
  http://www.nfpt.com

- **National Exercise Trainers Association (NETA)**
  http://netafit.org

- **National Association for Fitness Certification (NAFC)**
  http://www.nafctrainer.com

- **Aerobics and Fitness Association of America (AFAA)**
  http://www.afaa.com

- **National Exercise & Sports Trainers Association (NESTA)**
  http://www.nestapft.com

- **International Sports & Fitness Trainers Association (ISFTA)**
  http://isfta.com/about-us

- **Home Fitness Professionals Association (HFPA)**
  http://homefitnesspro.org

WEBSITES

- **National Strength and Conditioning Association (NSCA)**
  http://www.nsca-lift.org/Home

- **National Gym Association (NGA)**
  http://www.nationalgym.com

- **National Council on Strength & Fitness (NCSF)**
  http://www.ncsf.org

- **National Council for Certified Personal Trainers (NCCPT)**
  http://www.nccpt.com/User/Index.aspx

- **National Strength Professionals Association (NSPA)**
  http://nspacertified.com

- **National Fitness Trainers Association (NFTA)**
  http://www.nftafitness.com

- **IDEA Health & Fitness Association**
  http://www.ideafit.com

- **National Coalition for Promoting Physical Activity (NCPPA)**
  http://www.ncppa.org

- **International Fitness Professionals Association (IFPA)**
  http://www.ifpa-fitness.com

- **National Association for Health and Fitness (NAHF)**
  http://www.physicalfitness.org

- **Personal Trainer Today**
  http://www.personaltrainertoday.com

- **American Council on Exercise (ACE)**
  http://www.acefitness.org/aboutace
  /default.aspx

- **American Fitness Professionals & Associates (AFPA)**
  http://www.afpafitness.com

- **American College of Sports Medicine (ACSM)**
  http://www.acsm.org

EDUCATION WEBSITES

- **Raritan Valley Community College**
  http://www.rvccathletics.com/information/exerciseScience

- **Three Rivers Community College**
  http://www.trcc.commnet.edu/div_academics/admin
  /AS_Plans_of_Study/Assoc_Prog_of_Study_Webpage
  /Exercise%20Science_AS.shtml

- **Mesa Community College**
  http://www.mesacc.edu/programs/exercise-science

- **Washtenaw Community College**
  http://www.wccnet.edu/academics/programs/view
  /program/ASESCI/

- **University of Tampa**
  http://www.ut.edu/exercisescience

- **Mercy College**
  https://www.mercy.edu/academics/school-of-health-and-na
  tural-sciences/department-of-health-professions
  /bs-in-exercise-science

- **University of Massacusetts**
  http://www.umass.edu/ug_catalog/archive_2000/exsci.html

- **West Virginia University**
  http://majors.wvu.edu/home/details
  /231

- **Baylor University**
  http://www.baylor.edu/soe/hhpr/index.php?id=55755

- **Brigham Young University**
  http://exercisesciences.byu.edu/

- **University of Minnesota**
  http://www.cehd.umn.edu/future/undergraduate/majors
  /Kinesiology/default.html

- **Towson University**
  http://www.towson.edu/kinesiology

- **Kansas State University**
  http://www.k-state.edu/kines

- **Concordia University**
  http://excsci.concordia.ca

- **Broadview University**
  http://www.broadviewuniversity.edu/programs
  /health-science/health-fitness-specialist/personal
  -trainer-careers.aspx

www.ingramcontent.com/pod-product-compliance
Lightning Source LLC
Chambersburg PA
CBHW070941290526
45795CB00003B/1113